CANCER CURE

An essential guidebook on how to treat and prevent cancer

Dr Rowan Theo

Table of Contents

CHAPTER ONE

Curing Cancer: Treatments to Keep an Eye On

Cancer is a set of illnesses characterized through uncommon mobileular boom. These cells can invade exclusive tissues of the frame, main to extreme fitness problems.

most cancers is the second-main motive of loss of life in the United States at the back of coronary heart ailment.

Is there a remedy for most cancers? If so, how near are we? To solution those questions, it's critical to recognize the distinction among a remedy and remission:

• A remedy gets rid of all lines of most cancers from the frame and guarantees it won't come lower back.

• Remission approach there are few to no symptoms and symptoms of most cancers in the frame.

• Complete remission approach there aren't any detectable symptoms and symptoms of signs and symptoms of most cancers.

Still, most cancers cells can stay in the frame, even after whole remission. This approach the most cancers can come lower back. When this happens, it's generally in the first 5 years after remedy.

Some medical doctors use the term "cured" whilst regarding most cancers that doesn't come lower back inside 5 years. But most cancers can nonetheless come lower back after 5 years, so it's by no means honestly cured.

Currently, there's no actual remedy for most cancers. But latest advances in remedy and era are assisting pass us nearer than ever to a remedy.

Read directly to examine extra approximately those rising

remedies and what they might imply for the destiny of most cancers remedy.

Immunotherapy

Cancer immunotherapy is a kind of remedy that facilitates the immune machine combat most cancers cells.

The immune machine is made from numerous organs, cells, and tissues that assist the frame combat off overseas invaders, which includes bacteria, viruses, and parasites.

But most cancers cells aren't overseas invaders, so the immune machine might also additionally want a few assist figuring out them. There are numerous approaches of offering this assist.

Vaccines

When you observed of vaccines, you in all likelihood consider them in the context of stopping infectious illnesses, like measles, tetanus, and the flu.

But a few vaccines can assist save you — or maybe deal with — positive kinds of most cancers. For instance, the human papilloma virus (HPV) vaccine protects towards many kinds of HPV which could motive cervical most cancers.

Researchers have additionally been operating to expand a vaccine that facilitates the immune machine without delay combat most cancers cells. These cells regularly have molecules on their surfaces that aren't found in ordinary cells. Administering a vaccine containing those molecules can assist the immune machine higher apprehend and damage most cancers cells.

There's best one vaccine presently authorized to deal with most cancers. It's referred to as Sipuleucel-T. It's used to deal with superior prostate most cancers that hasn't spoke back to different remedies.

This vaccine is precise due to the fact it's a custom designed vaccine. Immune cells are eliminated from the frame and despatched to a laboratory in which they're changed so as to apprehend prostate most cancers cells. Then they're injected lower back into your frame, in which they assist the immune machine discover and damage most cancers cells.

Researchers are presently operating on growing and checking out new vaccines to each

save you and deal with positive
kinds of most cancers.

CHAPTER TWO

T-mobileular remedy

T cells are a sort of immune mobileular. They damage overseas invaders detected through your immune machine. T-mobileular remedy includes casting off those cells and sending them to a lab. The cells that appear maximum responsive towards most cancers cells are separated and grown in massive portions. These T cells are then injected lower back into your frame.

A precise kind of T-mobileular remedy is referred to as CAR T-mobileular remedy. During remedy, T cells are extracted and changed to feature a receptor to their surface. This facilitates the T cells higher apprehend and damage most cancers cells whilst they're reintroduced into your frame.

CAR T-mobileular remedy is presently getting used to deal with numerous kinds of most cancers, consisting of grownup non-Hodgkin's lymphoma and adolescence acute lymphoblastic leukemia.

Clinical trials are in development to decide how T-mobileular cures is probably capable of deal with different kinds of most cancers.

Monoclonal antibodies

Antibodies are proteins produced through B cells, every other kind of immune mobileular. They're capable of apprehend precise targets, referred to as antigens, and bind to them. Once an antibody binds to an antigen, T cells can discover and damage the antigen.

Monoclonal antibody remedy includes making massive portions of antibodies that apprehend antigens that have a tendency to be determined at the surfaces of most cancers cells. They're then injected into the frame, in which they are able to assist discover and neutralize most cancers cells.

There are many kinds of monoclonal antibodies which have been evolved for most cancers remedy. Some examples encompass:

• Alemtuzumab. This antibody binds to a selected protein on leukemia cells, concentrated on them for destruction. It's used to deal with continual lymphocytic leukemia.

• Ibritumomab tiuxetan. This antibody has a radioactive particle connected to it, permitting radioactivity to be brought without delay to the most cancers cells whilst the antibody binds. It's used to deal with a few kinds of non-Hodgkin's lymphoma.

• Ado-trastuzumab emtansine. This antibody has a chemotherapy drug connected to it. Once the antibody attaches, it releases the drug into the most cancers cells. It's used to deal with a few kinds of breast most cancers.

• Blinatumomab. This genuinely consists of exclusive monoclonal antibodies. One attaches to the most cancers cells, at the same time as the alternative attaches to immune cells. This brings immune and most cancers cells collectively, permitting the immune machine to assault the most cancers cells. It's used to deal with acute lymphocytic leukemia.

Immune checkpoint inhibitors

Immune checkpoint inhibitors raise the immune machine's reaction to most cancers. The immune machine is designed to connect overseas invaders with out destroying different cells in the frame. Remember, most cancers cells don't seem as overseas to the immune machine.

Usually, checkpoint molecules at the surfaces of cells save you T cells from attacking them. Checkpoint inhibitors assist T cells keep away from those checkpoints, permitting them to higher assault most cancers cells.

Immune checkpoint inhibitors are used to deal with numerous cancers, which includes lung most cancers and pores and skin most cancers.

Gene remedy

Gene remedy is a shape of treating ailment through enhancing or changing the genes in the cells of the frame. Genes incorporate the code that produces many exclusive sorts of proteins. Proteins, in turn, have an effect on how cells develop, behave, and speak with every different.

In the case of most cancers, genes end up faulty or broken, main to a few cells to develop out of manipulate and shape a tumor. The purpose of most cancers gene remedy is to deal with ailment through changing or editing this broken genetic facts with wholesome code.

Researchers are nonetheless reading maximum gene cures in labs or scientific trials.

CHAPTER THREE

Gene enhancing

Gene enhancing is a procedure for including, casting off, or editing genes. It's additionally referred to as genome enhancing. In the context of most cancers remedy, a brand new gene could be delivered into most cancers cells. This could both motive the most cancers cells to die off or save you them from growing.

Research remains in the early stages, however it's proven promise. So far, maximum of the studies round gene enhancing has worried animals or remoted cells, instead of human cells. But the studies is persevering with to strengthen and evolve.

The CRISPR machine is an instance of gene enhancing that's getting lots of interest. This machine lets in researchers to goal precise DNA sequences the usage of an enzyme and a changed piece of nucleic acid. The enzyme eliminates the DNA sequence, permitting it to get replaced with a custom designed sequence. It's sort of like the usage of the "discover and update" feature in a phrase processing application.

The first scientific trial protocol to apply CRISPR became currently reviewed. In the potential scientific trial, the investigators recommend to apply CRISPR era to adjust T cells in humans with superior myeloma, cancer, or sarcoma.

Virotherapy

Many kinds of viruses damage their host mobileular as a part of their existence cycle. This makes viruses an appealing ability remedy for most cancers. Virotherapy is using viruses to selectively kill most cancers cells.

The viruses utilized in virotherapy are referred to as oncolytic viruses. They're genetically changed to best goal and reflect inside most cancers cells.

Experts consider that once an oncolytic virus kills a most cancers mobileular, most cancers-associated antigens are released. Antibodies can then bind to those antigens and cause an immune machine reaction.

While researchers are searching at using numerous viruses for this kind of remedy, best one has been authorized so far. It's referred to as T-VEC (talimogene laherparepvec). It's a changed herpes virus. It's used to deal with cancer pores and skin most cancers which could't be surgically eliminated.

Hormone remedy

The frame obviously produces hormones, which act as messengers to the tissues and cells of your frame. They assist modify some of the frame's functions.

Hormone remedy includes the usage of a medicinal drug to dam the manufacturing of hormones. Some cancers are touchy to the degrees of precise hormones. Changes in those degrees can have an effect on the boom and survival of those most cancers cells. Lowering or blockading the quantity of a important hormone can gradual the boom of those kinds of cancers.

Hormone remedy is occasionally used to deal with breast most cancers, prostate most cancers, and uterine most cancers.

Nanoparticles

Nanoparticles are very tiny structures. They're smaller than cells. Their length lets in them to transport at some stage in the frame and engage with exclusive cells and organic molecules.

Nanoparticles are promising equipment for the remedy of most cancers, specially as a technique for handing over capsules to a tumor site. This can assist make most cancers remedy extra powerful at the same time as minimizing facet effects.

While that kind of nanoparticle remedy remains in large part in the improvement stage, numerous nanoparticle-primarily based totally shipping structures are authorized for the remedy of diverse kinds of most cancers. Other most cancers remedies that use nanoparticle era are presently in scientific trials.

How can opportunity remedy assist humans with most cancers?

Alternative most cancers remedies might not play an instantaneous position in curing your most cancers, however they will assist you address symptoms and symptoms and signs and symptoms because of most cancers and most cancers remedies. Common symptoms and symptoms and signs and symptoms consisting of tension, fatigue, nausea and vomiting, ache, problem sleeping, and strain can be lessened through opportunity remedies.

Integrating the first-class of evidence-primarily based totally complementary and opportunity most cancers remedies with the remedies you get hold of out of your physician might also additionally assist relieve some of the signs and symptoms related to most cancers and its remedy. Discuss all your alternatives together along with your physician and collectively you could decide which techniques may give you the results you want and that are probably to haven't any benefit.

Work carefully together along with your physician to decide the proper stability among conventional drugs and opportunity most cancers remedies. While complementary and opportunity most cancers remedies, consisting of acupuncture, might also additionally lessen nausea or ache, they usually are not effective sufficient to update most cancers medicinal drugs out of your physician.

Which opportunity most cancers remedies are really well worth trying?

These 10 opportunity most cancers remedies have proven a few promise in assisting humans with most cancers. Talk in your physician in case you're inquisitive about trying:

CHAPTER FOUR

• Acupuncture

. During acupuncture remedy, a practitioner inserts tiny needles into your pores and skin at particular points. Studies display acupuncture can be beneficial in relieving nausea because of chemotherapy. Acupuncture may assist relieve positive kinds of ache in humans with most cancers.

Acupuncture is secure if it is done through a certified practitioner the usage of sterile needles. Ask your physician for names of depended on practitioners. Acupuncture is not secure in case you're taking blood thinners or when you have low blood counts, so test together along with your physician first.

• Aromatherapy

. Aromatherapy makes use of aromatic oils to offer a chilled sensation. Oils, infused with scents consisting of lavender, may be carried out in your pores and skin all through a rubdown, or the oils may be brought to tub water. Fragrant oils also can be heated to launch their scents into the air. Aromatherapy can be beneficial in relieving nausea, ache and strain.

Aromatherapy may be done through a practitioner, or you

could use aromatherapy in your personal. Aromatherapy is secure, aleven though oils carried out in your pores and skin can motive allergic reactions. People with most cancers this is estrogen touchy, consisting of a few breast cancers, need to keep away from making use of massive quantities of lavender oil and tea tree oil to the pores and skin.

• Exercise.

Exercise might also additionally assist you control symptoms and symptoms and signs and symptoms all through and after most cancers remedy. Gentle workout might also additionally assist relieve fatigue and strain and assist you sleep higher. Many research now display that an workout application might also additionally assist humans with most cancers stay longer and enhance their general excellent of existence.

If you have not already been workout frequently, test together along with your physician earlier than you start an workout application. Start slowly, including extra workout as you go. Aim to paintings your manner as much as at the least half-hour of workout maximum days of the week.

• Hypnosis

. Hypnosis is a deep country of awareness. During a hypnotherapy session, a therapist might also additionally hypnotize you through speaking in a mild voice and assisting you relax. The therapist will then assist you attention on goals, consisting of controlling your ache and lowering your strain.

Hypnosis can be beneficial for humans with most cancers who're experiencing tension, ache and strain. It may assist save you anticipatory nausea and vomiting which could arise if chemotherapy has made you unwell in the past. When done through an authorized therapist, hypnosis is secure. But inform your therapist when you have a records of intellectual illness.

• **Massage.**

During a rubdown, your practitioner kneads your pores and skin, muscle tissues and tendons if you want to relieve muscle anxiety and strain and sell rest. Several rubdown strategies exist. Massage may be mild and mild, or it could be deep with extra pressure.

Studies have determined rubdown may be beneficial in relieving ache in humans with most cancers. It may assist relieve tension, fatigue and strain.

Massage may be secure in case you paintings with a informed rubdown therapist. Many most cancers facilities have rubdown therapists on staff, or your physician can refer you to a rubdown therapist who frequently works with humans who've most cancers.

Don't have a rubdown in case your blood counts are very low. Ask the rubdown therapist to keep away from massaging close to surgical scars, radiation remedy regions or tumors. If you've got most cancers for your bones or different bone illnesses, consisting of osteoporosis, ask the rubdown therapist to apply mild pressure, instead of deep rubdown.

CHAPTER FIVE

• Meditation.

Meditation is a country of deep awareness while you attention your thoughts on one image, sound or idea, consisting of a fantastic thought. When meditating, you may additionally do deep-respiration or rest sporting events. Meditation might also additionally assist humans with most cancers through relieving tension and strain.

Meditation is usually secure. You can meditate in your personal for a couple of minutes a couple of times an afternoon or you could take a category with an teacher.

• **Music remedy.**

During song remedy sessions, you may concentrate to song, play instruments, sing songs or write lyrics. A educated song therapist might also additionally lead you via sports designed to fulfill your precise needs, or you can take part in song remedy in a set setting. Music remedy might also additionally assist relieve ache and manipulate nausea and vomiting.

Music remedy is secure and does not require any musical skills to take part. Many clinical facilities have licensed song therapists on staff.

• Relaxation strategies

.   Relaxation strategies are approaches of focusing your interest on calming your thoughts and enjoyable your muscle tissues. Relaxation strategies may encompass sports consisting of visualization sporting events or revolutionary muscle rest.

Relaxation strategies can be beneficial in relieving tension and fatigue. They may assist humans with most cancers sleep higher.

Relaxation strategies are secure. Typically a therapist leads you via those sporting events and sooner or later you'll be capable of do them in your personal or with the assist of guided rest recordings.

• Tai chi.

Tai chi is a shape of workout that includes mild moves and deep respiration. Tai chi may be led through an teacher, or you could examine tai chi in your personal following books or videos. Practicing tai chi might also additionally assist relieve strain.

Tai chi is usually secure. The gradual moves of tai chi do not require excellent bodily strength, and the sporting events may be without difficulty tailored in your personal abilities. Still, speak in your physician earlier than starting tai chi. Don't do any tai chi movements that motive ache.

• Yoga.

Yoga combines stretching sporting events with deep respiration. During a yoga session, you function your frame in diverse poses that require bending, twisting and stretching. There are many kinds of yoga, every with its personal variations.

Yoga might also additionally offer a few strain comfort for humans with most cancers. Yoga has additionally been proven to enhance sleep and decrease fatigue.

Before starting a yoga class, ask your physician to propose an teacher who frequently works with humans with fitness concerns, consisting of most cancers. Avoid yoga poses that motive ache. A accurate teacher can provide you with opportunity poses which can be secure for you.

You might also additionally discover a few opportunity remedies paintings properly collectively. For instance, deep respiration all through a rubdown

might also additionally offer in
addition strain comfort.

THE END